Paleo **s**

MW00416199

Lose Weight And Get Healthy With These 30 Paleo Recipes

Introduction

I want to thank you and congratulate you for downloading the book, *"Paleo For Beginners - Lose Weight And Get Healthy With These 30 Paleo Recipes"*.

This book contains proven steps and strategies on how to adopt the paleo diet and lose weight.

Do you want to begin the paleo diet and are now looking for some delicious paleo recipes to incorporate into your diet? If you are, you need not look further: this book will provide you with 30 mouthwatering paleo recipes guaranteed to make your new paleo lifestyle a tasty.

When you follow the nutritional guidelines as directed by the paleo diet, you align yourself with evolutionary pressures, which shaped our current genetics. This is what in turn positively influences our health and wellbeing.

The diet lessens your body's glycemic load, contains an optimal balance of carbohydrates, fats, and proteins, and has a healthy ratio of saturated-to-unsaturated fatty acids.

Aside from the obvious benefit of weight loss, the paleo diet is also beneficial to digestion and absorption, a much healthier brain, healthier cells, reduced allergies, provision of necessary minerals and vitamins, improved gut health, and reduced risk of inflammation.

As you can see, the paleo lifestyle is a lifestyle worth adopting and using the 21 scrumptious paleo recipes in this guide, you can immediately start adopting the lifestyle.

Thanks again for downloading this book, I hope you enjoy it!

Table of Contents

Understanding Paleo

First things first, what is the paleo diet? The paleo diet is a diet solely based on foods our early ancestors used to eat during the Paleolithic era. The paleo diet is also known as the Stone Age diet, the primal diet, the hunter-gatherer diet, and the caveman diet. The diet operates on this simple tenet: what would a caveman eat?

This diet is one of the healthiest diets; as such, paleo enthusiasts do not consider it a diet per se – they consider it a lifestyle. It focuses on foods your Paleolithic ancestors supposedly consumed. These foods include meat, vegetables, seafood, nuts, and fruits.

Before we start discussing the diet, let us look at some important things you need to know about the diet:

As stated above, the paleo diet draws its tenets from this simple query: what would a Paleolithic man/our ancestors eat. As you may very well imagine, most of the foods that are today staples in our diets were not available during the Paleolithic era. As such, to understand and adopt the paleo diet, you need to understand which foods to eat and which ones to avoid. Let us look at that:

Paleo Dieting: Allowed Foods

When adopting the paleo lifestyle, here are the foods you can eat:

Nuts: Cashews, pecans, almonds, hazelnuts, macadamia nuts, walnuts, and pine nuts (moderate intake is necessary for weight loss)

Fresh fruits: watermelon, apples, pineapples, grapes, mango, avocado, lemon, strawberries, bananas, raspberries, lime, oranges, blackberries, peaches, plums, tangerine, papaya, figs, lychee, and blueberries (moderate your fruit intake)

Grass-fed meats: bacon, ground beef, pork chops, lamb rack and chops, bison rib eye, chicken wings, steak, ostrich, wild boar, turkey, goat, rattle snake, goose, clams, rabbit, reindeer, and kangaroo

Fresh vegetables: carrots, pumpkin, cabbage, peppers, cilantro, celery, mushrooms, cauliflower, butternut squash garlic, avocado, eggplant, peppers, radish, cucumber, spinach, zucchini, asparagus, shallot, onion, beets, and sweet potatoes

Healthy oils: coconut oil, avocado oil, macadamia oil, and olive oil

Fish/sea food: tuna, shrimp, crabs, sardines, tilapia, oysters, shark, sunfish, clams, salmon, trout, lobster, scallops, mackerel, Cray fish, halibut, swordfish, and walleye

Eggs

Paleo Dieting: Disallowed Foods

Avoid foods such as:
Candy
Processed foods
Refined vegetable oils
Legumes
Cereal grains
Dairy
Refined sugar
Overly salty foods

Potatoes

The Paleo Diet Rules

As stated, the paleo diet is Paleolithic in nature; as such, you should:

Think like a Hunter and Gatherer

This is the chief paleo diet rule. You probably should not eat any sort of food you could not hunt or gather back in the Paleolithic days. While on this diet, eat meat, veggies, fruit, and nuts.

Love Those Veggies

This diet emphasizes the consumption of lots of fresh veggies since meat was not always available to the early man. You get bonus points if you eat the ones local to your region and in season.

Cut Out the Processed Foods and Dairy

Since there were no domesticated cows in the early times, the early man could not have enjoyed an afternoon latte or the morning bowl of cereal with milk.

You also should avoid consuming any food that has an ingredients list of more than a single thing. The paleo diet highly discourages the ingestion of any processed food.

Workout Like a Caveman

Do not forget paleo workouts. The paleo diet, especially for weight loss and health purposes is not all about monitoring what you eat: you also <u>need</u> to exercise.

Incorporate exercises such as pull ups (like pulling yourself up to collect fruit from the top of a tree), short sprints (to simulate running from a dangerous wild animal such as a bear) and some other high intensity functional strength moves such as pushups, squats, and lunges to get the lean caveman look.

Catch the Meat Yourself or Choose Free-Range Meat

To experience the full paleo lifestyle, you can actually go out and hunt the meat yourself (of course following all laws and regulations). If you are not down for that, only opt for free-range, natural, and organic meat options. Your protein needs to remain as natural as possible.

Now that we have that out of the way, let us now look at tasty recipes

Paleo Breakfast Recipes

1. Mushroom Bacon Avocado Sandwich

Serves 1
Ingredients
2 thick slices avocado
2 Portobello mushrooms
½ lb. bacon
Several leaves of Lettuce (or some other type of greens)
Directions
1. Slice the bacon strips in halves, and then cook them covered to your liking.
2. Remove the bacon and leave it to drain on a plate.
3. Pour off most of the bacon grease (for later use) then return the pan back to the heat to keep hot.
4. Slice off the stem of the Portobello mushroom caps so that the whole cap is leveled and flat.
5. Place the Portobello mushroom caps in the bacon pan and cook for about 2 minutes on medium heat.
6. Place the cooked caps on a plate then stack the lettuce, avocado, bacon, and then top cap in that order.

2. Egg Muffins

Serves 12
Ingredients
12 eggs
1 tablespoon of olive oil
2 cups of spinach, chopped
1 chopped red bell pepper
1 cup of finely chopped mushrooms
¾ pound of nitrate-free ham slices
Salt and pepper to taste
Directions
1. Preheat your oven to 350 degrees Fahrenheit.
2. Heat the olive oil in a medium sized skillet. Lay two ham slices in each muffin tin while the olive oil heats up. To form a cup shape, press down the slices.
3. Once the oil is, add the bell pepper and mushrooms, and cook for a few minutes until the vegetables begin caramelizing and softening. Add the spinach to the now cooked vegetables and cook until just wilted.
4. Add a heaping spoonful of veggies atop the ham slices.
5. Crack an egg into the veggie and ham lined muffin tin.
6. Bake for around 12-15 minutes or until the egg whites cook through.
7. Remove from the oven and sprinkle with pepper and salt.

3. Pumpkin Spice Muffins

Yields 12 muffins
Ingredients
1 teaspoon of lemon juice
¾ teaspoon of baking soda
¼ teaspoon of ground cloves
½ teaspoon of ground ginger
1 teaspoon of ground cinnamon
6 eggs
¾ cup of maple syrup
½ cup of pumpkin puree
¾ cup of coconut flour
Directions
1. Preheat the oven to 350 degrees Fahrenheit.
2. Line a standard muffin tin with 12 silicone-baking cups or parchment paper.
3. Combine all the ingredients in a large mixing bowl and stir well with a whisk to break up any clumps.
4. Divide the batter into the 12 baking cups and bake for 25-30 minutes at 350 degrees Fahrenheit until the centers are firm and the edges are golden.
5. Let the muffins to cool in the pan for 10 minutes then transfer them to a wire rack to cool completely.
6. Place the muffins in sealed containers and store them in the fridge for 1 week or in the freezer for up to 6 months.

4. Sweet Potato Waffles

Yields 2
Ingredients
1/3 cup of almond milk
½ teaspoon of salt
1 cup of almond flour
½ teaspoon of nutmeg
2 tablespoons of coconut flour
2 eggs
½ teaspoon of baking soda
1 ½ teaspoons of vanilla
1 teaspoon of cinnamon
2 tablespoons of maple syrup
1 medium sweet potato, cooked and skin removed
½ tablespoon of coconut oil
Directions
1. Preheat the waffle iron
2. In a large bowl, mix all the dry ingredients.
3. In a separate medium bowl, whisk together all the other (wet) ingredients.
4. Pour the wet ingredients into the dry ingredients and mix until combined.
5. Pour the batter (since it will be thick, use a spatula to spread it out) onto the waffle iron and cook the batter in accordance with your waffle manual.

5. Apple and Bacon Sausage

Yields 14 to 18 patties
Ingredients
2 lbs. ground pork
Dash of cayenne powder
¼ teaspoon of ground cloves
1-2 teaspoons of sea salt (according to personal taste)
½ teaspoon of ground black pepper
½ tablespoon fresh lemon juice
1 tablespoon molasses (or honey, just a little less)
2 teaspoons of dried sage leaves (2 tablespoons of fresh chopped)
1 tablespoon of dried or fresh rosemary
1 medium apple, quartered and cored
¾ cup of chopped leeks (the white ends)
4-5 thickly cut strips of smoked bacon
Directions
1. Bake the bacon strips on a baking sheet for a few minutes at a temperature of 400 degrees Fahrenheit until they are about half way done.
2. Place all the ingredients apart from the pork into your food processor and process until everything is finely chopped.
3. Add the ground pork into the finely chopped mixture in the processor and pulse for only a couple of seconds until well mixed.
4. Throw a bit of the mixture into a pan and cook then taste to know if they require extra acid or salt before you make them into patties. Afterwards, make them into patties and place them on a baking sheet.
5. Bake for 30 minutes in the oven at 350 degrees Fahrenheit.

6. Shashuka

Serves 3
Ingredients
6 eggs
Salt and black pepper
2 tins of chopped tomatoes
1 pinch of saffron
2 teaspoons of smoked paprika
2 red peppers cut into strips
2 garlic cloves, finely chopped
1 onion, finely diced
1 tablespoon of fennel seeds
1 tablespoon of extra virgin oil
Finely chopped coriander
Directions
1. Heat the oil up then add the fennel seeds and leave them to cook for a minute.
2. Add the garlic and onion and cook for 3 more minutes.
3. Add the pepper, tomatoes, salt, spices and peppers and cook for 25 more minutes until the peppers become soft (add more water as you go).
4. Make some small wells on the tomato sauce then drop in the eggs and cover. Cook for another 5 minutes until the egg whites are cooked.
5. Serve with spinach.

7. Almond Flour Pancakes

Serves 2
Ingredients
2 large eggs
¼ teaspoon of sea salt
1 tablespoon of coconut oil, divided
¼ teaspoon of nutmeg, fresh
1 cup almond flour
¼ cup of water
½ cup of applesauce, unsweetened
½ cup of berries, fresh
1 tablespoon of coconut flour
Directions
1. Combine the eggs, applesauce, nutmeg, sea salt, almond flour and water in a bowl then mix them completely with a fork. The batter will appear thicker than normal mix.
2. Pour the coconut oil on a non-stick frying pan and heat it over medium-low heat.
3. Pour ¼ cup of the batter on the pan once it is fully heated. Slightly spread out the batter if desired.
4. When bubbles begin showing on the top, flip it like a normal pancake, then cook for one or two more minutes.
5. Add more oil to the pan and repeat the process with the remaining batter.
6. Serve and top with some fresh berries.

Paleo Lunch Recipes

8. Coconut Curry Chicken

Serves 6
Ingredients
¼ teaspoon of ground black pepper
1 teaspoon of fine-grain sea salt
2 tablespoons of arrowroot powder
1 teaspoon of chili powder
1 teaspoon of curry powder
2 teaspoons of garam masala
1 (170 grams) can of tomato paste
400ml can of full fat coconut milk
1 medium onion, chopped
3 minced garlic cloves
2 tablespoons of coconut oil
2lbs. free-range organic chicken breasts (cut into chunks)
Chopped coriander
Note: the arrowroot powder acts like the cornstarch
Directions
1. Heat the coconut oil in a medium skillet placed over medium heat.
2. Add the garlic and onion and sauté for 4 to 5 minutes or until translucent.
3. Add the chili powder, garam masala, and curry powder and sauté for 1 minute or until fragrant.
4. Stir in the pepper, salt, coconut milk, and tomato paste. Reduce the heat to low, add the arrowroot powder, and whisk until you see no lumps. Turn off the heat.
5. Use a bit of olive oil to grease the inside of your crock-pot bowl. Add the chicken chunks and pour the sauce all over them. Stir to coat.
6. Cover the crock-pot and cook on low setting for 5 hours.

7. Sprinkle the chicken chunks with chopped coriander before serving.

9. Spicy Roast Chicken

Serves 8

Ingredients

1/8 teaspoon of cayenne pepper

¼ teaspoon of paprika

¼ teaspoon of dried basil

¼ teaspoon of dried oregano

¼ teaspoon of ground black pepper

¼ teaspoon of salt

1 tablespoon of olive oil

1 (3 pound) whole chicken

Directions

1. Preheat your oven to 450 degrees Fahrenheit.

2. Thoroughly rinse the chicken both inside and outside under cold running water then remove all the fat. Use paper towels to pat the chicken dry.

3. Place the chicken in a small baking pan and rub it with olive oil.

4. Mix the cayenne pepper, paprika, basil, oregano, salt and pepper then sprinkle them over the chicken.

5. Roast the chicken in the preheated oven For 20 minutes. Lower the temperature to 400 degrees Fahrenheit and continue roasting for 40 more minutes to a minimum of an internal temperature of 165 degrees Fahrenheit.

6. Let the chicken to cool for 10–15 minutes then serve with your favorite dippings and vegetables.

10. Paleo Lasagna

Serves 4-6
Ingredients
For the beef and tomato sauce:
3 cups of tomato passata
2/3 teaspoon of sweet paprika
2/3 teaspoon of black pepper
3 garlic cloves, finely diced
2/3 cup of dry red wine
500g of grass-fed beef mince
1 teaspoon of ghee
1 ¼ teaspoon of sea salt
1 brown onion, diced
2 tablespoons of virgin olive oil
For the lasagna layers:
2-3 tablespoons of grated parmesan cheese (optional)
1 ½ cups of ricotta cheese (optional)
1 large eggplant, sliced into 1 cm-thick disks
2 teaspoons of ghee
3 zucchini, sliced vertically into thin ribbons
2 cups of baby spinach leaves
5-6 button mushrooms, sliced
½ cup of torn fresh basil leaves
1 large parsnip, peeled and sliced thinly
1 teaspoon salt
7 tablespoons virgin olive oil
Cherry tomatoes to garnish
Directions
1. Preheat your oven to 355 degrees Fahrenheit.
2. In a deep lasagna tray, place a layer of parsnip slices, a little ghee, and pre-bake in the oven for 15 minutes. This helps soften the layer slightly before building up the rest of the layers. Set it aside.

3. To make the sauce, cook the onion with some salt for 5-8 minutes (until it is slightly caramelized) and heat 2 tablespoons of olive oil.

4. Using a potato smasher or a spatula, stir and break the mince apart into small pieces since it tends to clump together during cooking. Cook until browned for 5-6 minutes.

5. To the cooking meat, add the following in the following order: red wine, pepper, salt, paprika, garlic, and fry for another 3-4 minutes. Add in the tomato passata, bring to a boil, turn down the heat to a simmering temperature, and cook for 10 minutes

6. Sprinkle sea salt on the eggplant slices and to draw out more juices, set aside for 10 minutes, rinse, and pat them dry. Reheat the oven back to 180 degrees Fahrenheit

7. Heat 1 tablespoon of ghee and 2 tablespoons of olive oil in a frying pan. Once hot, batch fry the eggplants for 2-3 minutes each side or until lightly golden browned. As you fry the eggplants, add more ghee and olive oil as needed. Set aside

8. Take out of the oven and layer the lasagna as follows : pre-cooked parsnips, ⅓ of tomato meat sauce, followed by eggplant slices, fresh basil leaves, then mushrooms, the meat sauce, spinach, zucchini, drizzle of olive oil and some cracked black pepper.

9. Cook for 35-40 minutes at 180 degrees Fahrenheit. If you are using grated Parmesan cheese and ricotta, add the two ingredients atop the lasagna at the 20 minutes cooking time mark.

10. In the last 10-15 minutes, increase the cooking temperature to 200 degrees Fahrenheit.

11. Garnish with cherry tomatoes and fresh basil.

12. Serve with a side mixed salad.

11. Chicken Stuffed Peppers

Serves 4

Ingredients

½ cup of fresh cilantro, chopped

4 medium yellow, red and/or orange sweet peppers

1 (14.5 ounce) can of no-salt added fire-roasted diced tomatoes

2 pounds of ground uncooked turkey or chicken

2 tablespoons of Mexican seasoning (find recipe below)

1 medium Serrano chile or jalapeno, chopped and seeded

4 cloves of garlic, minced

½ cup of chopped onion

2 tablespoons of extra virgin olive oil

Lime wedges

For the Mexican seasoning (makes about ¼ cup):

¼ teaspoon of ground saffron

½ teaspoon of ground cinnamon

4 teaspoons of paprika

½ to 1 teaspoon of ground cayenne pepper or chipotle pepper (optional)

1 teaspoon of dried oregano

1 tablespoon of granulated garlic, preservative-free

1 tablespoon of cumin seeds

Directions

1. Heat the oil over medium heat in a large skillet.

2. Add the chile, garlic and onion then cook and stir for 2 minutes.

3. Add the ground chicken and cook until it is no longer pink.

4. Sprinkle with the Mexican seasoning and stir well.

5. Stir in the un-drained tomatoes in the mixture and bring to boil. Reduce the heat and simmer uncovered until most of the liquid evaporates for around 5-7 minutes. Stir the ¼ cup of cilantro in the mixture.

6. Cut the sweet peppers vertically in half. Remove and do away with the membranes, seeds, and stems. Blanch the peppers in boiling water in a large pot until tender for around 2-3 minutes. Drain and fill the peppers with the chicken mixture.

7. Arrange 2 pepper halves on a plate for each serving. Sprinkle with the rest of the cilantro then serve with the lime wedges.

8. *For the Mexican seasoning:* toast the cumin seed in a small dry skillet for 1-2 minutes over medium-low heat, shaking the skillet occasionally. Remove from the heat and cool for 2 minutes. Place the seeds in the spice grinder and grind them to a powder. Transfer the cumin to a small bowl then stir in the chipotle pepper (if using), saffron, oregano, paprika, cinnamon and garlic. Place in an airtight container at room temperature for up to 6 months. Shake or stir before use.

12. Picadillo Lettuce Wraps

Serves 4-6
Ingredients
For the picadillo:
2 tablespoons of drained capers
1 teaspoon of freshly ground black pepper
2 tablespoons of green olives with pimiento, diced
¼ cup of currants
1 (14 oz) can of whole tomatoes
2 tablespoons of olive brine (or salt and white wine vinegar)
½ teaspoon of ground cinnamon
1 teaspoon of ground cumin
½ teaspoon of salt
1 large green pepper, diced
1 medium onion, diced small
2 tablespoons of coconut oil, lard or tallow
1 pound of grass-fed ground beef
For the pico de Gallo:
Salt to taste
2 teaspoons of fresh lime juice
2 tablespoons of minced cilantro
2/3 cups of diced tomatoes
1/3 cup of minced red onion or shallot
To serve
Chopped cilantro (optional)
Cabbage leaves or lettuce leaves
Directions
1. Heat a Dutch oven or a large skillet over medium heat. Add the beef then crumble and stir occasionally during the cooking. Remove and set aside.
2. Add oil or tallow to the pan then add the onions and cook them until they begin to soften (takes around 3-4 minutes).

3. Add the bell pepper and cook for another 3 minutes. Add in the garlic and stir then add the cumin, cinnamon, black pepper and the salt and stir until fragrant for 30 seconds.
4. Add the currants, capers, canned tomatoes, olive brine, diced olives and cooked beef. While the mixture comes to a boil, break the tomatoes up into small pieces.
5. Reduce the heat to low then cover and simmer for around 10-20 minutes.

For the pico de Gallo: combine the minced cilantro, dash of salt, minced shallot, limejuice and chopped tomatoes then set aside.

To serve, fill each of the lettuce leaf with a spoonful of the beef mixture and a spoonful of cilantro or the pico de Gallo.

13. Baked Tilapia with Radish

Serves 4

Ingredients

1 tablespoon of lemon juice

2 tablespoons of drained capers, chopped

1 green onion, trimmed and finely chopped

1 bunch of trimmed and finely chopped radishes

½ lemon, very thinly sliced crosswise

1/8 teaspoon of black pepper, freshly ground

1/8 teaspoon of fine sea salt

4 (8 ounce) boneless and skinless tilapia fillets

Directions

1. Preheat your oven to 400 degrees Fahrenheit.

2. Cut parchment paper into 4 (12 inch) squares. Fold each of the square parchment paper in half so that you can form a crease at the middle then unfold it. On each piece of paper, place one tilapia fillet ensuring you arrange it just to one side of the crease. Top the fillets with the lemon slices, pepper, and salt.

3. Fold the parchment paper over to cover the fish completely. To seal the pouches, fold in the corner and edges until all the open sides are secure.

4. Transfer the sealed pouches to a baking sheet and bake for 10 minutes or until the fish cooks through.

5. For the relish, combine the lemon juice, capers, radishes, and green onion.

6. Place each of the sealed pouches on an individual plate to serve. Carefully use scissor to snip an opening at the top then peel back the paper and evenly divide the radish relish among the plates.

Paleo Dinner Recipes

14. Paleo "Spaghetti" with Meat Sauce

Serves 4
Ingredients
1 teaspoon of dried oregano
Salt and pepper
Extra virgin olive oil for drizzling
1 spaghetti squash
For the sauce:
Salt and pepper to taste
1 tablespoon of Italian seasoning
½ jar of tomato sauce
1 tomato, chopped
1 tablespoon of coconut oil
4 cloves of minced garlic
1 small onion, chopped
1 lb. ground beef or turkey
Fresh basil, for garnish
Directions
1. Preheat your oven to 400 degrees Fahrenheit.
2. Cut the squash in half lengthwise. Scoop the seeds out and discard.
3. Place the squash halves with the cut side up on a rimmed baking sheet. Drizzle with olive oil and season with oregano, salt, and pepper.
4. Place the squash in the oven and roast for around 40-45 minutes until you can easily poke with a fork.
5. Let the squash to cool until you can handle it safely. Use a fork to scrape the insides of the squash to shred it into strands.
6. As the spaghetti squash cooks, melt the coconut oil in a skillet over medium heat. Add the garlic and the chopped onion and leave them to cook for 4-5 minutes.

7. Add the ground turkey and let the meat to brown remembering to stir occasionally. Season the meat with pepper and salt.

8. Add the Italian seasoning, chopped tomato, tomato sauce, and then stir to combine. Simmer on low heat (while stirring occasionally).

9. Serve over the spaghetti squash with basil for garnish.

15. Crab Cakes with Lemon Vinaigrette

Serves 4
Ingredients
Vinaigrette:
1 teaspoon of raw honey, warmed if solid
½ teaspoon of garlic powder
½ teaspoon of onion powder
1 teaspoon of prepared ground mustard
½ teaspoon of lemon zest
3 tablespoons of fresh squeezed lemon juice
½ cup of extra virgin oil
Crab cakes:
4 tablespoons of lard/bacon tallow, or fat (for cooking the crab cakes)
1/3 cup of almond flour (plus a little extra for dusting)
1/8 teaspoon of cayenne pepper
1 teaspoon of sea salt
½ teaspoon of garlic powder
1 ½ teaspoon of yellow prepared mustard
1/3 cup of paleo mayonnaise
1 large egg, whisked
2 tablespoons of fresh squeezed lemon juice
½ cup of yellow and red bell pepper, chopped small
1/3 cup of green onion, chopped
1 pound lump of crab meat
Salad:
1 lemon, quartered (for serving)
6 cups of rinsed and dried arugula
Directions
1. To make the dressing, whisk all the vinaigrette ingredients until well blended then put in the fridge until you are ready to serve

2. *To make the crab cakes:* in a large mixing bowl, place all the ingredients and very gently mix until fully combined. If the mixture is too wet, add a little more of the almond flour. Shape the mixture into cakes and dust them lightly with additional almond flour.

3. Over medium high heat, heat the bacon fat/lard or tallow in a large skillet and let the fat to get hot.

4. Cook the crabs in batches for around 3-5 minutes on each side until browned. Ensure you turn them gently and carefully once during cooking.

5. Place the batch on a plate covered with paper towels and finish cooking the remaining crab cakes. Serve immediately.

6. To assemble, place a cup of arugula on the plate then top with 2-3 crab cakes. Drizzle some of the vinaigrette over the crab cakes, and then serve with a lemon wedge.

16. Smoked Lamb with Grilled Asparagus

Serves 8

Ingredients

1 lemon, cut into quarters

¼ teaspoon of black pepper

1 tablespoon of olive oil

2 bunches of fresh asparagus

2 tablespoons of snipped fresh thyme

1 ½ teaspoons of black pepper

 2 tablespoons of finely shredded lemon peel

2 tablespoons of coriander seeds

1 (2-3 pound) boneless leg of lamb

1 cup of hickory wood chips

Directions

1. Soak the hickory chips in a bowl with enough water to cover then set them aside.

2. Meanwhile, over medium heat, toast the coriander seeds in a small skillet for about 2 minutes until fragrant and crackling, stir frequently. Remove the cooked coriander seeds from the skillet and leave to cool.

3. Coarsely crush the seeds in a mortar and pestle after they have cooled or place them on a cutting board and use the back of a wooden spoon to crush them.

4. Combine the lemon peel, thyme, crushed coriander seeds, and the 1 ½ teaspoons of pepper in a small bowl and set aside. If the netting is present on the lamb roast, remove. Open up the roast on a work surface, fat side down.

5. Sprinkle half of the mixture of spices on the meat and use your fingers to rub it in.

6. Roll up the roast then tie it with 4-6 pieces of cotton kitchen strings. Sprinkle the outside of the roast with the remaining mixture of spice, pressing lightly to stick.

7. Arrange the medium-hot coals around a drip pan for a charcoal grill; test whether the heat is medium above the pan. Sprinkle the now drained wood chips all over the coals. Place the lamb leg over the drip pan on a grill rack.

8. Cover the meat and leave to smoke for around 40-50 minutes for a medium of 145 degrees on a meat thermometer. (If you are using a gas grill, preheat the grill then reduce the heat to medium. Adjust the grill to indirect cooking and smoke as explained above except you should add the drained wood chips depending on the directions of the manufacturer). Lightly cover the roast in a foil and leave it to stand for 10 minutes before slicing it up.

9. Meanwhile, you could be trimming the woody ends from the asparagus. Toss the asparagus with the ¼ teaspoon of black pepper and the olive oil in a large bowl.

10. Place the asparagus perpendicular to the grill grate and directly over the coal around the outer edges of the grill.

11. Cover them and leave to grill for around 5 to 6 minutes until they are crisp tender.

12. Squeeze the lemon wedges all over the asparagus and remove the string from the lamb roast. Thinly slice the meat and serve with the grilled asparagus.

17. Paleo Beef Enchiladas

Serves 4
Ingredients
9 paleo tortillas
3 tablespoons of fresh cilantro, chopped
1 avocado, diced
1 jalapeno, minced
½ onion, finely diced
2 tablespoons of extra virgin olive oil, divided
1 lb. ground beef
For the sauce:
Salt to taste
¼ teaspoon of dried oregano
½ teaspoon of cumin
2 tablespoons of chili powder
2 cups of chicken broth
2 cups pureed tomatoes
4 garlic cloves, minced
1 small onion diced
Directions
1. Heat 1 tablespoon of olive oil over medium-low heat in a heavy saucepan to make the enchilada sauce. Sauté the garlic and onion for 4-5 minutes until soft.
2. Add the rest of the ingredients apart from the salt and bring to a boil. Reduce the heat and let it simmer for 15-20 minutes until the sauce becomes thick. Season with the salt to taste.
3. If you wish, you could use an immersion blender to puree the garlic and onion into the sauce.
4. Meanwhile, in a large skillet, heat a tablespoon of olive oil over medium heat.

5. Add the onion to the oil and sauté for 4-5 minutes or until soft. Stir in the jalapeno and ground beef then season with pepper and salt; cook until the meat looks brown then remove from the heat. To coat the meat, stir in a few spoonfuls of the enchilada sauce.

6. Preheat your oven to 350 degrees Fahrenheit.

7. Coat the bottom of a 9 x 13 inch baking dish with a very thin layer of the enchilada sauce. Fill each of the tortillas with the meat mixture, roll over, and then place them side by side in the baking dish.

8. Cover them with the remaining enchilada sauce and bake for 12-15 minutes.

9. Serve immediately topped with cilantro and avocado.

18. Butternut Squash Soup

Serves 6
Ingredients
3 cups of chicken broth
2 tablespoons of ghee
1 teaspoon of chili powder
½ teaspoon of cumin
1 ½ teaspoons of salt
2 teaspoons of cinnamon
3 tablespoons of olive oil
2 carrots chopped
1 small yellow onion, chopped
1 green apple, cored and sliced
1 large butternut squash, cubed
Directions
1. Preheat your oven to 400 degrees Fahrenheit.
2. Combine the cumin, salt, cinnamon, olive oil and the butternut squash in a large bowl and mix them together, coating the squash well. Spread the butternut squash on a rimmed baking sheet
3. Toss the apple slices, carrots, and onions in the bowl that had the squash to coat with the remnants.
4. Place the mixture on a second rimmed baking sheet then place both sheets in the oven. Roast until soft for 35-40 minutes stirring once.
5. Heat up the ghee in a large pot on the stove over medium heat. Add in the roasted ingredients then the chicken broth. Add 1 teaspoon each of chilli powder, salt and cinnamon. Bring them to a boil and reduce the heat to low then simmer uncovered for 20 minutes.
6. Use an immersion blender to blend then serve warm.

19. Paleo Mini Meatloaf

Yields 18 mini meatloaves

Ingredients

¼ teaspoon of nutmeg

1 teaspoon of dried thyme

1 teaspoon of garlic powder

2 teaspoons of onion powder

2 teaspoons of pepper

2 teaspoons of salt

1/3 cup of coconut flour

4 eggs, lightly beaten

2 carrots, finely diced or grated

6 ounces of mushroom, finely diced

1 medium onion, finely diced

1-2 teaspoons of oil

10 ounces of frozen chopped spinach

2 pounds of ground meat – a mixture of grass-fed beef and/or veal and/or pork

Directions

1. Preheat your oven to 375 degrees Fahrenheit.

2. Thaw the spinach then squeeze out the excess water and set aside.

3. Heat your pan over medium heat and add the oil then fry the mushrooms and onions until some of the liquid in the mushroom has cooked out and the onions are translucent. Set aside to cool.

4. In a large bowl, place the ground meat then add the mushroom/onion mixture, coconut flour, carrots, beaten eggs, all the spices and the spinach. Combine it well with your hands but don't over mix.

5. Pour the meatloaf mixture in 18 regular size muffin tins and fill them to the top. (if you are using fairly lean meat, grease the tins).

6. Serve the meatloaves with vegetables and homemade sauce.

Paleo Dessert Recipes

20. Chocolate Brownies

Serves 12
Ingredients
2 ½ tablespoons of coconut flour
1 teaspoon of baking soda
1 teaspoon of baking powder
½ cup of raw sifted cacao powder
2 teaspoons of vanilla extract
1/3 cup of honey
½ cup of melted coconut oil
2 whole eggs
1 medium sweet potato (makes 2-3 cups when grated)
Directions
1. Preheat your oven to 365 degrees Fahrenheit (ensure the oven is hot before you place in the brownies).
2. In a large mixing bowl, combine the coconut oil, grated sweet potato, vanilla, honey, eggs, and stir together until well incorporated.
3. Add the baking soda, baking powder, and cacao powder. Do not add to much coconut flour since it will absorb too much moisture, which will result in drier brownies.
4. Once fully combined, pour the mixture into the baking tray lined with greased baking paper.
5. Bake for 25-30 minutes, remove the tin and leave to cool for 5-10 minutes before you carefully remove the brownie cake from the tin.
6. Cut the brownie cake into squares and dust with a little cacao or you could melt some dark chocolate in a microwave or over boiling water then drizzle it over the top of the brownies.

7. Serve with some strawberries or raspberries, and maybe coconut yoghurt.

21. Berry Ice Cream

Serves 8

Ingredients

½ teaspoon of vanilla extract

2 cans of full fat coconut milk

1 pinch of salt

½ cup of maple syrup

2 ½ cups of fresh mixed berries (blueberries, raspberries)

Directions

1. Combine the salt, berries, and maple syrup in a medium pot then bring to a boil.

2. Reduce the heat to a gentle simmer then cook for 3-4 minutes until the berries begin to burst. Remove from the heat and leave them to slightly cool.

3. Add the vanilla extract, coconut milk, and the berry mixture to a blender and process until smooth and creamy.

4. Pour the blended mixture into an ice cream maker and leave to freeze according to the manufacturer's instructions.

5. You could serve immediately or transfer to a covered container then store in the freezer.

6. Before serving, ensure you leave the ice cream to thaw in the refrigerator for around 20 to 30 minutes.

22. Almond Bars

Serves 2

Ingredients

1/3 cup of coarsely chopped almonds
3 tablespoons of agave nectar
A pinch of salt
¼ teaspoon of vanilla bean paste
1/3 cup of coconut sugar
½ teaspoon of almond flour
2 cups of unsweetened coconut
1/3 cup of cocoa powder
¼ cup of melted coconut oil
2/3 cup of softened coconut butter
¾ cup of almond butter

Directions

1. Line an 8 × 8 inch glass-baking dish with parchment paper and lightly grease the bottom and sides with coconut oil.
2. Whisk together the salt, coconut powder, vanilla bean paste, coconut oil, almond butter, and coconut sugar. This will make the crust of the bars.
3. Press the crust mixture firmly into the prepared baking pan then place it in the refrigerator while you begin preparing the second layer.
4. For the second layer, place the coconut in a medium sized mixing bowl then set it aside. Whisk together the agave nectar, almond flavoring, and coconut butter in a separate bowl.
5. Pour your coconut butter mixture over the coconut then mix well.
6. Retrieve the pan from the refrigerator and press the second layer onto the first layer. Top with the chopped almonds. If desired, you may drizzle ganache over the bars.
7. Place the two layered bar back into the refrigerator and leave until they are completely set.

23. Caramel Cheesecake Bars

Serves 24
Ingredients
For the crust:
½ cup of dates, pitted
¼ teaspoon of salt
1 cup of blanched almond flour
For the cheesecake:
1 teaspoon of vanilla extract
½ cup of raw honey
½ cup of coconut oil
1 teaspoon of lemon juice (optional)
½ cup of coconut oil
12 oz. raw cashews soaked for 1 to 2 hours, then drained
For the caramel:
1 teaspoon vanilla extract
5 tablespoons of canned full fat coconut milk
3 tablespoons of filtered water
Pinch of salt (plus extra for the top)
20 dates, pitted and soaked for an hour then drained
Directions
1. Place the crust ingredients inside the food processor and mix until smooth.
2. Press the smooth crust mixture into a 8×8 inch brownie pan.
3. Wipe out the food processor then add all the ingredients for the cheesecake and pulse until smooth.
4. Spread over the cooled crust mixture then freeze again as you prepare the caramel.
5. Place the caramel ingredients inside the food processor and process for about 3 minutes.
6. Spread the caramel mixture over the cheesecake layer then place the pan back inside the freezer.
7. Cut the cheesecake into squares after 30 minutes. If there are any leftovers, store them back in the freezer.

24. Paleo Donuts

Yields 12 mini donuts
Ingredients
Donuts:
½ cup of warm apple cider
2 tablespoons of honey
2 tablespoons coconut oil (liquid)
2 eggs (at room temp)
1/8 teaspoon of celtic sea salt
½ teaspoon of baking soda
½ teaspoon of cinnamon
2 tablespoons of ghee (or coconut oil) melted for coating the cooked donuts
½ cup of coconut flour
Cinnamon sugar:
1 tablespoon of cinnamon
½ cup of granulated coconut sugar
Directions
1. Preheat your donut maker.
2. Whisk together the cinnamon, coconut flour, salt and baking soda in a small bowl.
3. In another medium bowl, whisk the honey, oil, and eggs.
4. Add the whisked dry ingredients into the whisked wet ingredients then stir until combined.
5. Add warm apple cider to the mixture and mix until it is incorporated into the dough fully.
6. Scoop the donut batter and place it in the preheated donut maker (a cookie scooper will make it easy). Use about 1 ½ tablespoons for each donut.
7. Close the lid and cook for around 2-3 minutes
8. Remove the cooked donuts from the donut maker carefully. You could either brush the donuts with melted coconut oil/ghee to cover both sides.

9. Toss the donuts in the cinnamon/coconut sugar mixture you prepared until coated.

Paleo Snacks and Smoothies

25. Guacamole

Yields 2 ½ cups
Ingredients
2 tablespoons of fresh lime or lemon juice
½ cup of chopped cilantro
½ white onion
1 firm tomato, diced finely
3 medium avocados or 4 small ones
Optional salt and pepper to taste
Directions
1. Cut open the avocados and scoop out the flesh.
2. Use a fork to mash the flesh. You may still leave hard parts – do it according to your preference.
3. Stir in the rest of the ingredients.
4. You could enjoy it right away with some paleo crackers or store it in the refrigerator. Place a plastic wrap that will touch the guacamole to prevent it from browning due to contact with air.

26. Butternut Chips

Serves 4
Ingredients
Pinch of salt
1 teaspoon of gingerbread spice mix (1/2 teaspoon of cinnamon, pinch of cloves, allspice, nutmeg, and ginger)
2 tablespoons of ghee or extra virgin coconut oil or red palm oil, melted
1 medium butternut squash (400g)
Optional: 3-6 drops of liquid stevia extract
Directions
1. Preheat your oven to 250 degrees Fahrenheit.
2. Peel the butternut squash then use a mandolin to slice it thinly. If you are using a knife, ensure that the slices are not more than ¼ cm (1/8 inch) thin. Place the slices in a bowl.
3. In a small bowl, mix the stevia, gingerbread spice mix, and melted coconut oil.
4. Pour the oil mixture all over the butternut squash then mix it well to ensure it is everywhere.
5. Arrange the slices close to each other on a rack or an oven chip tray (you will require at least two of them) or on a baking tray lined with parchment paper.
6. Place them in the oven and cook for 1.5 hours or until crispy (the specific time depends on how thick you make your chips).
7. You should keep an eye on the chips even though they should not burn when cooked at low temperature.
8. When done, leave them to cool then store them in an airtight container for up to a week.

27. Avocado Smoothie

Serves 2

Ingredients

2 cups of coconut or almond milk

1-2 tablespoons of unsweetened cocoa powder

½ cup of frozen raspberries (or just fresh berries)

2 frozen bananas

1 avocado

Directions

1. If your frozen bananas are not peeled, remove them from the freezer and leave them to thaw for 10 minutes before you peel them.

2. Place all the ingredients in the blender and blend them well.

28. Paleo Mango Smoothie

Serves 1

Ingredients

½ teaspoon of pure vanilla extract

Honey (optional – depending on how sweet your mango is)

Ice

3 tablespoons of freshly squeezed orange juice

1/3 cup of full fat coconut milk (or almond milk)

½ cup of frozen or fresh mango

Directions

1. Place all the ingredients in a blender or a single serve mixture.

2. Blend until just creamy then serve.

29. Pumpkin Pie Smoothie

Serves 2

Ingredients

1/8 teaspoon of cinnamon (plus 1/8 teaspoon more to garnish

1/8 teaspoon of allspice

1/8 teaspoon of nutmeg

1/8 teaspoon of ginger

¼ teaspoon of vanilla extract

1 teaspoon of maple syrup

1 ½ cups of almond milk, unsweetened

½ cup of pumpkin puree

1 ½ frozen bananas

Directions

1. Place all the ingredients in the blender (except for the reserved cinnamon for garnishing) and blend on high until smooth.

2. Pour the smoothie in a glass then garnish with the cinnamon and enjoy.

30.   Strawberry Coconut Smoothie

Serves 2

Ingredients

1 teaspoon of frozen vanilla extract

2 cups of frozen strawberries

1 frozen banana sliced

1 cup of coconut milk

Directions

1. Pour all the ingredients in a high-speed blender and blend until smooth.

Conclusion

Thank you again for downloading this book!
I hope this book was able to help you to learn about the paleo diet, the foods you can eat, those to avoid and some recipes to get you started.
The next step is to adopt the diet and enjoy the amazing results it has to offer.

Finally, if you enjoyed this book, would you be kind enough to leave a review for this book on Amazon?

Click here to leave a review for this book on Amazon!

Thank you and good luck!

Check Out My Other Books

Below you'll find some of my other popular books that are popular on Amazon and Kindle as well. Simply click on the links below to check them out. Alternatively, you can visit my author page on Amazon to see other work done by me.

- Juicing for Beginners Secrets To The Heathy Benefits of Juicing 30 Unique Recipes

If the links do not work, for whatever reason, you can simply search for these titles on the Amazon website to find them.

92546531R00030

Made in the USA
Columbia, SC
28 March 2018